Acting Edition

I0741561

Sleeping Giant

by Steve Yockey

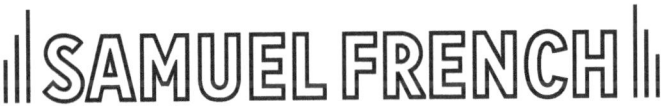

MUSIC AND THIRD-PARTY MATERIALS USE NOTE

IMPORTANT BILLING AND CREDIT REQUIREMENTS

SLEEPING GIANT received its world premiere at Salt Lake Acting Company (Cynthia Fleming, Executive Artistic Director) in North Salt Lake City, Utah, on September 21st, 2022. The production was directed by Emilio Casillas and Shawn Francis Saunders, with scenic design by Halee Rasmussen, lighting design by Jessica Greenberg, costume design by Bett Shouse, sound design by Cynthia L. Kehr Rees, props design and construction supervision by Erik Reichert, and projection design by Michael Francis. The EDI Dramaturg was Latoya Cameron. The Production Stage Manager was Jennie Sant. The cast was as follows:

THE NAÏF . . . . Lily Hye Soo Dixon
THE RACONTEUR . . . . Robert Scott Smith
THE MESSENGER. . . . . .Tito Livas
THE CONVERT . . . . Cassandra Stokes-Wylie

SLEEPING GIANT was originally produced by Mark Giberson, Nathan Frizzell, Michael Matthews, and Christopher Sepulveda as part of the Edinburgh Festival Fringe 2019. The performance was directed by Michael Matthews. The cast was as follows:

THE NAÏF . . . . Katie Skelton
THE RACONTEUR . . . . .Adam Silver
THE MESSENGER. . . . . Rick Cosnett
THE CONVERT . . . . Daisy Eagane

SLEEPING GIANT was commissioned by Theater Emory in Atlanta, GA, for their "4:48 Project" and received additional development through Center Theatre Group's L.A. Writers' Workshop Festival.

CHARACTERS

TRACK 1 – The Naïf

ALEX

MAGGIE

JESSIE

MULTITUDES

ZEALOT

TRACK 2 – The Raconteur

RYAN

PATRICK

NATHAN

DAN

TRACK 3 – The Messenger

BILLY

HIDDEN MAN

GUS

CHARLIE

BUTTERFLY KING

TRACK 4 – The Convert

BARBARA

JILL

MABEL

MULTITUDES

AUTHOR'S NOTES

[ ] in the script indicate overlapping dialogue.

Licensees should retain the doubling outlined in the Character Breakdown as the doubling is specific to the storytelling.

This all moves swiftly, careening ahead. The attention is on the individual stories. Let the background events loom and grow.

All of this takes place in the living rooms of different homes – except for Scene Six, which takes place in some mythic place. The shadow puppetry called for in this scene can be live, pre-recorded, or accomplished through animation. Ideally any solution will maintain the stylistic qualities of shadow puppetry.

One
Miasma

(A living room of a lake house. Night. Fireworks can be heard offstage, but very close. Too close and exceedingly loud. The colorful pops and glows of the firework explosions spill into the space through windows.)

*(Some smoke seeps in and then **RYAN** and **ALEX** enter through it, coughing a bit. He's excited. She's a lot less excited.)*

RYAN. That was amazing!

ALEX. I can't breathe!

RYAN. Wasn't [that amazing?!]

ALEX. [Jesus, Ryan, I can't] [breathe!]

RYAN. [Just give it] a second. It's only the smoke, it'll be fine in a second.

ALEX. Ryan.

RYAN. That was so, that was even more massive than I planned. There were some really big guys mixed in there I didn't even know about.

(He claps with excitement, but is also still coughing.)

ALEX. Fuck you.

RYAN. Oh, come on!

*(**ALEX** walks over and slaps at **RYAN** repeatedly.)*

ALEX. Are you trying to get us killed?! What in the hell is wrong with you setting [off all of those fireworks like that?! Are you crazy?!]

RYAN. [Alex, Alex, stop it. Ouch, Alex, calm] down!

ALEX. Don't you tell me to calm down. You scared me to death!

(He's still amused. She is not.)

RYAN. It was supposed to be a surprise.

ALEX. Surprise, you're on fire and now you're dead from shock.

RYAN. You didn't think it was a little bit beautiful?

ALEX. I know it was a lot illegal. And that was way bigger than just store-bought fireworks.

RYAN. Yep! Isn't it fun?

(He coughs.)

ALEX. Where did you even get those massive fireworks? That was, like, some industrial-level shit.

RYAN. But did you think it was beautiful?

ALEX. I'm not going to, I'm not ready to concede that point yet because I can still taste that awful smoke in the air.

RYAN. I'm gonna take that as a "yes."

ALEX. I will pack a bag.

RYAN. You know you loved it.

ALEX. I will go upstairs and pack my bag right now and leave this lake house. You think I'm dying to sleep on your mother's old mattress? I don't care how good the sex is or how nice [the view is...]

RYAN. [Hold up, hold] up, Alex. What's wrong with my mother's mattress?

ALEX. I can feel. The springs. In my back.

RYAN. [It's not that bad.]

ALEX. [And god knows what kind] of dust and mites and little, invisible things are all over it after years of being [in the woods.]

RYAN. [Excuse me,] your highness.

ALEX. You almost blew us up!

RYAN. Are you really upset?

ALEX. Yes I'm really upset!!

RYAN. But you love fireworks.

ALEX. No, fireworks scare the shit out of me. You love fireworks. And you love seeing how they freak me out. And you thought this would be fun for you and used me as an excuse to do it and honestly that's par for the course.

RYAN. Whoa.

ALEX. You're not allowed to say, "Whoa." I'm still saying "Whoa." Like, "Whoa, I cannot believe he doesn't get it."

RYAN. I didn't realize you felt that way.

(She sees that she landed a blow and softens.)

ALEX. I mean, I'm sure my reaction is a little oversized because I'm freaked out, but yes, I feel that way. Sometimes.

RYAN. Then...you don't want the second part of your surprise?

ALEX. Oh god, there's more.

RYAN. Yes.

ALEX. But the air is still thick and smoky from the first part.

> (**RYAN** *takes a small box out of his pocket and takes a knee. He opens the box, revealing a lovely wedding ring.*)

Are you fucking kidding me?

RYAN. Nope.

ALEX. Get up.

RYAN. Alex, I have loved you since the first day [we met.]

ALEX. [Get up.]

RYAN. We've been through thick and thin and, honestly, we both know that no one else in the world could put up with either of us.

ALEX. Do we though?

RYAN. And I am sure that, even though you're pissed at me right now, I should one hundred percent be your husband. Will you marry me?

> (**ALEX** *coughs some more.*)

And I'm sorry about the smoke.

ALEX. I'm deaf now from the explosions. Ask me again.

RYAN. Will you marry me?

ALEX. Probably.

RYAN. Probably?

ALEX. That's right, probably. First, explain why you did this?

> (*He gets up, but he's still holding the ring box out.*)

RYAN. Oh, sure. So I've been reading this really fascinating book called, *Lost Palace of The Butterfly King*.

ALEX. And?

RYAN. And it's really good.

ALEX. There needs to be more to the story.

RYAN. Oh, so the book is an excavation of this weird ancient religion in the South Pacific that worshipped Blue Moon butterflies. And they had all these crazy rituals. One of them was specifically a marriage thing, or their version of marriage, which was lovely and had flower crowns and a naked swim in the river. But then it was also kind of gruesome and involved cutting up and eating the father-in-law.

ALEX. Ryan!

RYAN. I know, it's bizarre, right?

ALEX. It's cannibalism.

RYAN. The cannibalism was just for marriages. Or actually for a lot of occasions, they killed themselves, they killed each other, I guess it's whatever the "Butterfly King" wanted.

ALEX. The Butterfly King wanted death and cannibalism?

RYAN. It doesn't matter, just forget that part.

ALEX. Oh, just forget about the part where they kill and eat [each other?]

RYAN. [Yes, because] before any of that, when a man wanted to marry a woman, he would do this dance, this like ecstatic dance, and then ignite this huge bonfire to let everyone in the village know he was intending to wed.

ALEX. And then they would swim naked in the river?

RYAN. Yes.

ALEX. And eat people.

RYAN. We agreed to forget about that part.

ALEX. And so the fireworks are your bonfire declaration?

RYAN. Well actual bonfires are illegal around the lake.

ALEX. So are fireworks!

RYAN. I hear you and I respect your concerns. So are you ready to say, "yes" yet?

ALEX. Where's my dance?

RYAN. What?

ALEX. In your horrific butterfly book, [you said...]

RYAN. [*Lost Palace*] of *The Butterfly King*.

ALEX. You said the man did an "ecstatic dance" and then lit a bonfire. So where's my dance? Did I miss it?

RYAN. You want a dance?

ALEX. Absolutely.

RYAN. You don't think I will? Fine. Here, will you take this thing, please?

>   (**ALEX** *takes the ring box.*)

Ha! You took the ring.

ALEX. Dance.

>   (*He proudly, dramatically takes his shirt off.*)

Okay.

>   (**RYAN** *starts to jump around. It's a sort of mix of dancing, sexy posing, and bad mime. It's joyful and silly and very sweet.*)

>   (**ALEX** *lets it go on for a while.* **RYAN** *stops. He is breathing heavy.*)

That was definitely ecstatic.

RYAN. Dance. Bonfire. Proposal. So...?

(RYAN walks over, grabs the ring box, opens it, and kneels again. She takes the ring and puts it on.)

ALEX. You are ridiculous. And the fireworks were maybe a tiny bit beautiful.

RYAN. I love you, too.

(He gets up and they kiss.)

And we'll stop with the traditions there. No one has to eat anyone.

ALEX. And now we go swim naked in the river?

RYAN. It's a lake house. There is a lake. But you do have to be okay with sleeping on my mother's mattress because it's the only one in the house.

ALEX. Deal.

(They kiss again, more passionately. But the kiss is interrupted by the sound of a loud, high-pitched roaring from somewhere in the distance. It's far away, but unsettling. It also has an odd, rumbling reverberation. They're both a bit unnerved by the noise.)

RYAN. What was that?

ALEX. I've never heard anything [like it.]

RYAN. [Oh! Oh! Maybe] it was the Butterfly King celebrating our engagement?

ALEX. Enough.

RYAN. You don't know what the Butterfly King sounds like.

ALEX. Is this a South Pacific Island? Okay, I changed my mind about the marriage [thing now.]

RYAN. [Too late!] You're stuck with me.

ALEX. We didn't do the cannibalism part, so officially I can still back out.

> (**BILLY** *tumbles in. He's barefoot, wearing jean shorts and a gray T-shirt with a vintage "1976" emblazoned on it. He's out of it. Dazed, but amped up. Almost manic. He's bleeding from the nose.)*

> (**ALEX** *and* **RYAN** *are clearly startled and confused.)*

RYAN. What the fuck?!

ALEX. Billy?

RYAN. You scared the shit out of us.

BILLY. I didn't, what are you, what?

RYAN. Billy, this isn't your house. You're in the wrong house.

BILLY. Nobody, nobody's home at my house.

ALEX. He seems really [out of it.]

RYAN. [Is something] wrong? Are you okay?

> (**RYAN** *puts his shirt back on.)*

ALEX. Oh! Oh, he's bleeding. His nose is, do you need help?

BILLY. Yes, I don't know, um, [it was, it was...]

ALEX. [Billy, you're] bleeding, are you hurt? Did something happen to you?

> (**BILLY** *touches his nose and looks at the blood on his fingers. It's not reflective though, he doesn't calm down.)*

BILLY. I was, I was standing by the lake and it had just got dark and then someone set off fireworks or something, but like really close, too close.

(**ALEX** *and* **RYAN** *share a look.*)

It was so loud, the water actually shook, it shook.

RYAN. So I have a confession to [make about…]

BILLY. [And then] it, and then it happened. It opened.

RYAN. What?

BILLY. I saw an eye open. There was something in the lake, in the water, something alive and it opened its eye.

RYAN. Like a fish?

BILLY. Bigger, bigger than a fish.

RYAN. How much bigger?

BILLY. And it had these arms, not arms, tentacles, a lot of them, too many. It seemed, I think the fireworks maybe woke it up. And it smelled like something died, muddy and rotting, you know that smell in the air?

ALEX. Okay, I see, I get it, you didn't like the fireworks. I didn't like them either. But Billy, we just got engaged and you're wrecking it with this prank.

BILLY. You got, what?

RYAN. Just now. We set off fireworks. I did, that was me. They were supposed to go higher, but I didn't really know what I was doing and [the smoke…]

BILLY. [But it's not] a prank! It's not a prank and I can prove it!

ALEX. Okay, try to calm down.

BILLY. I took a picture, I took a picture and when the flash went off, the pupil sort of got tight or, like, zeroed in. And it was right there. It was so close, just below the surface of the water, even though the lake is deep along there, right? But it was like it had been there forever. And the eye was, you asked me how big, my friend Mike was with me, he was standing next to it and the eye alone was the size of his, of his whole body.

RYAN. Wait, Mike was with you?

(He looks at his hand.)

BILLY. So I reached out and...and I touched the eye.

ALEX. Billy, where is Mike? Is he okay? [Is he...?]

BILLY. [No, no he's] not. And I touched the eye and then it made this noise, this crazy loud noise, and the water glowed, I know how that sounds, but it glowed with this pale light as far as I could see, and the thing tilted up out of the water and I've never, it was just...

(He's shaking a bit.)

It was larger than anything I've ever seen.

ALEX. Okay, Ryan, he's freaking me out.

RYAN. Billy, are you on, did you take something?

ALEX. You should, he should go, right? Can you ask him to go?

RYAN. If no one's at your house, is there, can we call someone for you?

BILLY. I can still feel it on my hand. I can still hear it on my hand. And it made a noise like this...

(He opens his mouth and the high-pitched roaring sound from earlier comes out of his mouth. Deafeningly loud now, it fills the entire space. **RYAN** *and* **ALEX** *scream out, covering their ears.)*

*(***BILLY*** closes his mouth and the roar stops. They all stand in an uneasy silence. What was that?)*

Who do...who do you call for that?

Two
Eyeball

*(A different suburban living room. **MAGGIE** waits patiently on a couch. She is dressed for an upscale brunch. Chic with a chunky necklace or something. She seems cool. **BARBARA** is talking to **MAGGIE** from somewhere out of sight.)*

*(There is a **HIDDEN MAN** standing in the corner of the room. A dark figure facing the corner.)*

MAGGIE. You can't see me, but I'm looking at my watch.

BARBARA. *(Offstage.)* I'm sorry, I know. Also, you don't wear a watch.

MAGGIE. Barbara, we are two single, busy women. Brunch with the girls is one of our few perks. And you know there's going to be a line if we don't hurry. Personally, I don't want to wait in line for those pancakes. I will wait in line, but I don't want to.

BARBARA. *(Offstage.)* Thank you so much for your patience. I'm trying something new and it's turning out to be more of a project than I ever imagined.

MAGGIE. That doesn't sound good.

BARBARA. Oh, but I really think you're going to love it. You know how you're always telling me to be more adventurous?

MAGGIE. I don't think I've ever said that.

BARBARA. *(Offstage.)* Oh, you know, like how you've encouraged me to try new things.

MAGGIE. I said we shouldn't eat at the same restaurant every Sunday. Mostly because I'm manipulative and wanted to try these peach pancakes.

BARBARA. *(Offstage.)* Well I extrapolated what you said into a larger mission.

MAGGIE. That's not what I intended. But if you're happy then I'm sure...

> (**MAGGIE** *stops short as* **BARBARA** *enters. She's in a skirt and blouse. Chic. Notably, she's wearing a small fascinator on her head with a single, enormous peacock or pheasant feather protruding out of it. Honestly, it seems to defy gravity.)*

BARBARA. I'm ready.

MAGGIE. Oh wow.

BARBARA. What?

MAGGIE. That hat.

BARBARA. It's not a "hat." It's a fascinator.

MAGGIE. Okay.

BARBARA. The milliner says there's a difference.

MAGGIE. Okay.

BARBARA. And I'm assuming that the milliner who owns a hat shop knows more about millinery than you or I do, ostensibly.

MAGGIE. And you go to a milliner now?

BARBARA. I went to a milliner. Is that so unusual?

MAGGIE. Yes, Barbara.

BARBARA. Well, I don't know about that, and I only went the one time, but you absolutely cannot get something like this in a department store.

MAGGIE. Department stores sell hats.

BARBARA. It's not a hat.

MAGGIE. Did it...did it come in a hatbox?

BARBARA. Yes.

MAGGIE. I mean...

(**MAGGIE** *shrugs as if to say, "I guess it's a hat."*)

BARBARA. The milliner said there's a difference.

MAGGIE. Okay, this is just eating up time. So let's just agree it's a bold fashion statement and get going.

HIDDEN MAN. Eyeball.

BARBARA. I think it's bold, too. Oh no, are you being sarcastic?

MAGGIE. Absolutely not, I [wouldn't...]

BARBARA. [I think you're] being sarcastic.

MAGGIE. I would never be sarcastic about your...fascinator.

BARBARA. Thank you.

(**MAGGIE** *grabs her purse and stands to go.* **BARBARA** *is all smiles but doesn't move. She almost looks confused.* **MAGGIE** *stands to go.* **MAGGIE** *waits as the silence piles up.*)

(**MAGGIE** *sits back down. What is going on?*)

MAGGIE. Do you want to talk about it?

BARBARA. I just thought I'd try something different.

MAGGIE. Not the hat.

BARBARA. Fascinator.

MAGGIE. Do you want to talk about whatever's going on with you that has you acting so odd?

BARBARA. But I'm perfectly fine.

MAGGIE. Okay, we won't talk about it.

BARBARA. I'm not being at all evasive.

MAGGIE. Fine, we'll do it the slow way. So you went to the hat store?

BARBARA. That's right.

MAGGIE. I've known you for most of my life and I've never seen you wear a hat.

BARBARA. Well observed.

MAGGIE. So does this have something to do with the crying?

> (**BARBARA** *laughs nervously.*)

BARBARA. What crying?

MAGGIE. Barbara, you don't have to do that. Because ever since I found you crying in your kitchen the other day you've really been working overtime to try to convince me that you're not upset about [anything.]

BARBARA. [But I'm] not upset.

HIDDEN MAN. Eyeball.

> (**BARBARA** *visibly winces at the sound of the word.*)

MAGGIE. Look, not to be reductive, but in our friendship, I am the adventurous one and you are the down to earth one. But that hat [really does...]

BARBARA. [Fascinator.]

MAGGIE. That thing on your head screams, "Something is wrong." So won't you just tell me what's going on with you? And then we can go get yummy peach pancakes. Because I think that massive feather on your head is a call for help. Or you're trying to fly, which is not [going to work.]

BARBARA. [Well, maybe I] am trying to fly.

MAGGIE. It's not going to work.

HIDDEN MAN. Eyeball.

> (**BARBARA** *visibly winces again. She's trying to hide it. How long has this been going on?*)

BARBARA. Okay, okay, we can talk about it. You win. But let's not talk about it here. Let's talk about it at brunch, I feel bad for making [you wait.]

MAGGIE. [But we] have privacy here?

BARBARA. All right.

MAGGIE. Good. We've already waved goodbye to a spot in line. And I can't one hundred percent tell, but this seems like something we should discuss here as opposed to in front of a bunch of hungry brunchers.

> (**BARBARA** *leans in, momentarily desperate, and whispers...*)

BARBARA. Are you very sure we can't just go to brunch?

MAGGIE. Oh my god, stop acting weird and talk to me.

BARBARA. I'll do my best.

> (*Suddenly, everything goes dark as pink specials zero in on* **BARBARA** *and the* **HIDDEN MAN**. *They are the only things illuminated onstage now. And the lights seem to undulate on them, oily and odd.*)

> (**BARBARA** *begins to quietly sing a version of the children's nursery rhyme "Three Blind Mice." But it's choked and breathy, as if she's being forced to do it. A version of* **BARBARA***'s voice comes from elsewhere, singing the song sweetly along with her. The difference is disconcerting.*)

(The **HIDDEN MAN** *whistles along with* **BARBARA***, still facing away from the audience. His whistle might even be amplified. This entire moment is eerie, and it lasts. It happens outside of time.* **MAGGIE** *isn't frozen, per se. She's simply not present for this.)*

BARBARA.

THREE BLIND MICE, THREE BLIND MICE,
SEE HOW THEY RUN, SEE HOW THEY RUN,
THEY ALL RAN AFTER THE FARMER'S WIFE,
WHO CUT OFF THEIR TAILS WITH A CARVING KNIFE.
DID YOU EVER SEE SUCH A THING IN YOUR LIFE,
AS THREE BLIND MICE?

(When they finish the tune, it hangs in the air a moment. But now everything is very quiet and **BARBARA** *looks terrified.)*

(Then the lights abruptly shift back to normal and it all resumes. **MAGGIE** *is still waiting for* **BARBARA** *to continue.)*

MAGGIE. Barbara?

BARBARA. I said I'll do my best. To tell you. But it's a ridiculous story. Fair warning. So my friend's son was up at the lake, and he took a picture of something. Something very odd. I don't know how to describe it. I guess it was sort of like a Loch Ness monster photo because it really [can't be real.]

MAGGIE. [He photographed] the Loch Ness monster here?

BARBARA. Not the Loch Ness monster, but like that. He took a photo of something in the lake, something very large and very alive.

MAGGIE. So like a fish?

BARBARA. Not like a fish. Much, much larger. His friend is in the photo, so it kind of creates a sense of scale and it's so much larger than you could...

MAGGIE. Barbara?

BARBARA. Yes? Yes, so in the photo you can see this thing's eye. Staring at him. He showed me the photo himself. And it was unsettling. I was, he had to hold my hand. I'm not usually, you know me, I don't have time for that kind of nonsense. But I found the photo very upsetting and he squeezed my hand. And we just looked at it. And ever since, I'm feeling out of sorts.

MAGGIE. Okay, I'm trying to follow you here. You were crying in your kitchen because of the photo?

BARBARA. I mean, yes. But it's more than that.

> (*The* **HIDDEN MAN** *begins to visibly breathe heavier. We can even hear him. It's menacing.* **BARBARA** *smiles again. Tight and intense.*)

MAGGIE. Jesus, why is it like pulling teeth to get you to talk about it?

BARBARA. It only feels like that because I don't want to talk about it.

MAGGIE. Well, you should talk to me about it because this isn't, oh my god, Barbara, why are you breathing so heavy? You are not having a normal reaction to seeing some hoax picture of a lake monster.

> (**BARBARA** *suddenly leans in again and grabs* **MAGGIE**'*s hand. She speaks in a seething whisper.*)

BARBARA. That's because it wasn't a normal thing.

MAGGIE. Barbara! You're hurting my hand.

BARBARA. It isn't a hoax, I looked at the picture and the eyeball, in the picture, the eyeball moved, it moved, that thing looked at me from the photo, it just –

*(The **HIDDEN MAN** suddenly screams at the top of his lungs, cutting **BARBARA** off. It is punctuated, harsh, and unsettling. **BARBARA** covers her ears, but **MAGGIE** doesn't seem to notice.)*

MAGGIE. Barbara, what is wrong with you?

BARBARA. You didn't hear that?

MAGGIE. I didn't hear anything.

*(**BARBARA** smiles again. Intense.)*

BARBARA. I'm fine. I'm just being silly, you're sweet to worry, but I'm fine.

MAGGIE. You are not fine. I'm your best friend and you are not fine.

BARBARA. You are my best friend.

MAGGIE. I know.

BARBARA. You trust me, don't you?

MAGGIE. Of course I do.

BARBARA. I can tell you don't like the fascinator.

MAGGIE. Barbara!

BARBARA. The fascinator just makes me feel confident. It's like an anchor, it just makes [me feel...]

MAGGIE. [Barbara, I don't] give a fuck about the goddamn hat. You are coming unhinged, I'm sorry to be blunt, but you need some help.

BARBARA. Because of the fascinator?

MAGGIE. Okay, we are going to get you some help.

BARBARA. I don't want you to miss the peach pancakes.

MAGGIE. Are you serious?

HIDDEN MAN. Eyeball.

BARBARA. Oh my god.

MAGGIE. Will you please let me take you somewhere right now? Because I'm not going to leave you when you're frankly acting crazy.

HIDDEN MAN. Eyeball.

(**BARBARA** *tries to respond to* **MAGGIE**, *but instead all she can say is...*)

BARBARA. Eyeball.

MAGGIE. What?

BARBARA. Eyeball?

MAGGIE. Why are you saying that?

(**BARBARA** *reaches for* **MAGGIE**'s *hand again, but* **MAGGIE** *pulls away. It legitimately seems like this is the only word* **BARBARA** *can say now.*)

(*The* **HIDDEN MAN**, *still facing the corner, raises his hands up above his head and shakes his arms wildly. It's disconcerting.*)

BARBARA. Eyeball. Eyeball. Eyeball! Eyeball! [Eyeball!]

MAGGIE. [Stop it! Stop] it or I'm leaving! Barbara, [I am serious.]

(**BARBARA** *leaps up from the coach, her body stiff, fists clenched tightly, and starts shouting!*)

BARBARA. [Eyeball!] Eyeball! Eyeball! [Eyeball!]

MAGGIE. [Please, Barbara,] [you're scaring me.]

BARBARA. [Eyeball! Eyeball!] Eyeball! Eyeball! Eyeball! Eyeball! Eyeball!

(It goes on and on. **MAGGIE** *gets up and backs away, but* **BARBARA** *shows no intention of stopping.* **MAGGIE** *rushes out.)*

(Eventually **BARBARA** *stops. She stands there in shock, breathing heavy. The* **HIDDEN MAN** *stops shaking his hands and lowers them.)*

*(***BARBARA** *tries to calm down. Is it over? After a moment...)*

HIDDEN MAN. Eyeball.

*(***BARBARA** *starts crying.)*

Three
Cuckoos

*(Another living room. **MABEL** is in jeans and a T-shirt or blouse. Also a fun little apron. It's an "at home cook" kind of thing. She carries a cake into her living room. It's lovely. She sets the cake down and admires it. Suddenly there's a pounding on the door that startles her!)*

MABEL. Oh! Oh my god. Who is it?

GUS. It's Gus. I'm out here with Patrick. Open up!

*(**MABEL** lets **GUS** and **PATRICK** inside.)*

MABEL. You guys, you scared me. I'm in the middle of something. Can it wait?

PATRICK. We literally rushed over here.

MABEL. And you can go to your home and come back later when I'm not busy.

GUS. You have to hear what Patrick has to say. We need, like, we need your, I don't know, you're just better at dealing with stressful shit.

MABEL. I know you didn't just swear in my house.

GUS. I'm [sorry.]

PATRICK. [He's sorry,] Mabel.

MABEL. Now is whatever you're going to tell me bad? Because I'm in a really Zen place and I just baked a cake, so I don't [want to...]

GUS. [I'm not] messing around, Mabel, this is important.

MABEL. Okay, okay. But let me go get some more plates for the cake since you're here and all.

GUS. We don't need cake!

MABEL. Nobody "needs" cake. Is someone dying? If someone's not dying right now then I'm getting some plates. Just hold on two seconds.

> *(She exits. The **BOYS** are still catching their breath.)*

PATRICK. She is gonna flip out.

GUS. I'm flipping out.

PATRICK. I mean it's a big deal, it's huge.

GUS. Yeah. What is that smell?

> *(**MABEL** comes back with some small plates and a serving knife.)*

MABEL. I burned something. I'm sorry. I wasn't expecting anyone. Okay, tell me.

GUS. Did you see the video of the people by the lake?

MABEL. So this is bad.

GUS. Mabel.

MABEL. I don't want to talk about those people or their violence down by the lake.

GUS. Fine, but just did you see the video?

PATRICK. Because I saw something in the lake. Like in person, I think I saw it. Or I'm kind of sure I saw it because there's no other explanation.

MABEL. You saw it in real life?

> *(**PATRICK** tells his story. **GUS** "helps." They are talking fast and bringing a lot of energy. This story will be familiar to readers as the Book of Revelation. But for our purposes, it's the quick, chaotic story of the crazy thing Patrick saw at the lake. It is not recited with any kind of deliberate awe or biblical grandeur.)*

PATRICK. So this was before people started talking about it and I didn't say anything because I didn't think anyone would believe me. But I went out there one night a while back. I went out there to the lake and I stood on the sand of the lake, I stood on the sand and I saw something.

MABEL. What did you see?

PATRICK. It was a beast.

GUS. It was a beast!

MABEL. A beast?!

PATRICK. Yes! I saw a beast rise up out of the water.

MABEL. So it is real?

PATRICK. Yes. I saw a beast rise up from the water, having seven heads!

MABEL. Wait, "having seven heads?"

PATRICK. And ten horns!

GUS. That's right! Ten horns!

PATRICK. And upon his horns ten crowns!

GUS. One for every horn!

PATRICK. Yes!

MABEL. Why are you using such, I don't know, archaic [language?]

PATRICK. [And upon each] head was written the name of blasphemy.

MABEL. Oh dear.

PATRICK. And the beast which I saw was like unto a leopard.

MABEL. "Like unto?"

GUS. It looked like a leopard.

MABEL. Ah.

PATRICK. And his feet were as the feet of a bear.

MABEL. What?

GUS. Yeah, he told me.

PATRICK. And his mouth as the mouth of a lion.

MABEL. Wait, what?

PATRICK. And the dragon gave him his power, and his seat, and great authority.

(**MABEL** *is scandalized!*)

MABEL. There was a dragon?

PATRICK. And everyone wondered after the beast.

GUS. They wondered after the beast!

MABEL. Wondered?

PATRICK. [Wondered!]

GUS. [Wondered!]

MABEL. Well, there has been a lot about it on television and [in the papers.]

PATRICK. [And they] worshipped the beast.

MABEL. Who? The people by the lake?

GUS. [Yes!]

PATRICK. [Yes!] And they all said, "Who is like unto the beast? Who is able to make war with him? [Who is like unto the beast?"]

GUS. ["Who is like unto the beast?"]

MABEL. Oh no.

PATRICK. And there was given unto him a mouth, an enormous mouth, for speaking great things and blasphemies against God.

MABEL. Oh no, this is, this is, you saw all of this?

PATRICK. Yes. Why?

MABEL. It's just so much.

PATRICK. Yes.

GUS. It is so much.

MABEL. But I had heard on the news earlier that people were saying it looked like a gigantic glowing squid or something.

PATRICK. They did?

MABEL. Yes.

PATRICK. Were there pictures?

MABEL. Not that I've seen.

PATRICK. Then I'm sticking with it looked like a leopard.

GUS. With bear feet and a lion mouth.

MABEL. Well, you have to trust your own eyes.

PATRICK. Right? And because of the Bible.

MABEL. I'm sorry?

PATRICK. Because that's the description in the Bible. In the Book of Revelations. When they're talking about how the world ends and there's a beast with all [of those...]

GUS. [I thought] you said you saw it?

PATRICK. I did.

GUS. When you told me this story you didn't say anything about the Bible.

PATRICK. Look, I went out there and I got high and I saw something and then there were all these reports on the news about weird things, so I inferred it.

MABEL. From what you saw? When you were high?

GUS. So you did or did not see this thing?

PATRICK. Well...not directly.

GUS. Not directly? You've got me over here repeating this stuff, probably freaking Mabel out, and now [it's "not directly?"]

PATRICK. [I maybe just, I] was just trying to make sense out of it a little bit, I'm scared, it's [scary, okay?]

GUS. [So you're scaring] other people?

(**MABEL** *steps in.*)

MABEL. Both of you listen. It's all right to be scared. This is an unsettling time. Honestly, I've been scared too.

GUS. Yeah?

MABEL. Between us? I'm terrified every morning when I wake up. It's terrifying. But I realized, and maybe it's good you came over after all, because I realized three things that have really helped me find some peace about all of this uncertainty. And potential horror.

(*She nods knowingly.*)

PATRICK. So come on then, Mabel?

GUS. Will you tell us?

MABEL. Yes. Yes, I will. Here, have some cake. What I'm going to say is comforting, I promise, but it might sound a little bleak at first and everything is better with cake.

(*As she speaks, she cuts a slice of cake for each of them and herself. Once handed out, they all eat as she shares her thoughts.*)

Now who knows if any of these stories are real? But let's say they are, for the sake of argument. The world has been around for a long time. Who knows how long that thing has been in that lake? Or wherever it was before we stumbled on it. It shouldn't exist, but it does. It survived. Some creatures do and some creatures don't.

GUS. Natural selection.

MABEL. That's right, Gus. And frankly, the verdict is still out on us. Not just us three, the verdict is still out on people in general. Maybe, if we're lucky, we're like sharks and we just keep going? Or maybe we're like dinosaurs and we just get the time we get? Or maybe we're like cuckoo birds and we just keep singing the same two soothing notes over and over while the world falls apart around us? But ultimately looking at the big picture of the waves of life on this planet kind of helps gain a little perspective.

PATRICK. Because everything ends?

GUS. Except sharks.

MABEL. Even sharks will end. And if our time is up and weird giants are taking over then that's just how it is. If you consider it that way, it makes it less about us specifically, doesn't it? And another thing, if it turns out the stories about this "beast" are true, about what it can do to people, then that doesn't mean it's the end. We can adapt. That's something we've been doing for a long time. Adapting. Evolving. Dealing with change. We're good at it. Some of us are good at it anyway. So there's hope. Or there's cake. In light of all that, it can't really be all that awful.

(She takes a bite.)

PATRICK. You're right. And the cake is very good.

MABEL. Thank you.

GUS. Still warm.

MABEL. Well I iced it too soon, but it's holding up okay. Anyway, doesn't all that make you feel at least a little better? Not better, but calmer.

PATRICK. Yes. But you only said two of the things?

MABEL. I'm sorry?

GUS. You said you figured out three things to feel better and you only said two of the things. Or did I miss the third one?

PATRICK. Right, the dinosaurs and how we adapt to things.

MABEL. And the cake.

PATRICK. Oh, the cake. Okay.

GUS. I didn't realize the cake was the third thing. Sorry.

MABEL. Don't apologize. Like I said, some of us are good at adapting. I'm not. I know that about myself. So when I saw that video of those people at the edge of the lake dancing, praying almost, cutting themselves, cutting their own throats and throwing themselves into the water. Or it was dark, but it seemed like that's what they did. I thought, "I don't know what to do with this. If this is real, where do I put this?"

PATRICK. Yes, that's it exactly.

MABEL. So for a few days I experienced what I imagine was some form of existential crisis or psychotic break, I don't know, it was pretty awful. And then I burned most of my personal belongings in the basement. That's the smell. I turned off all the smoke alarms, but I think the smoke actually got in the walls.

GUS. Mabel, why did you burn your things?

MABEL. Because nothing means anything anymore.

GUS. Oh wow.

MABEL. I told you it was bleak. Anyway, then I baked this cake. With a lot of foxglove. Do you know it?

GUS. No?

MABEL. It's a plant. It's full of an extremely poisonous substance called digitoxin that causes paralysis, I guess, and more likely cardiac arrest. In fact, I baked this cake so full of foxglove it's sure to paralyze my diaphragm and suffocate me in minutes now if I don't have a heart attack first.

> *(***GUS** *and* **PATRICK** *look at the cake they've been eating.)*

And honestly either of those things feels better than this new, unknown world. It's all too much. I don't want to know any more things. Oh, and I'm so glad I got to share this with you. Cakes are made for sharing.

Four
Ginger & Wasabi

*(Another living room. **JILL** enters her home with a plastic bag in hand. She looks like she just came from yoga. Or that's just how she dresses.)*

JILL. Nathan? I'm back.

*(Just as she's setting down her purse, **NATHAN** enters. He's rubbing either side of his nose. He's in jeans and some band T-shirt. Casual.)*

NATHAN. Hey.

JILL. That was amazing. Hardly any traffic. I mean people are not out and about, where is everyone?

NATHAN. I didn't even know you left.

JILL. You were doing the neti pot.

NATHAN. Oh wow, I didn't wait for it to cool down. I think I scalded my brain.

JILL. Pouring hot water in your nose will do that.

NATHAN. Make fun all you want, but if you tried it then you'd never go back.

JILL. I'm fine. I breathe fine, thanks. Did it help?

NATHAN. All cleared out. So you ran an errand?

JILL. Remember I told you my sister is coming over?

NATHAN. No. Which one?

JILL. Jessie.

NATHAN. Ah, the "older" one.

JILL. What was that? What does that mean?

NATHAN. You know what it means. It means that most of the time, older sisters are the responsible ones. But your older sister is...not that. So I put "older" in air quotes.

JILL. Well, quit it.

NATHAN. Am I wrong?

JILL. She called and told me that she's bringing over some special health food thing for us to try. Well, she was more cryptic. You know how she is, but anyway it's something like that. And I was supposed to invite Mabel too, but she hasn't been answering her phone all day. So it's just us.

NATHAN. Mabel would have baked something nice to eat at least.

JILL. Something unhealthy.

NATHAN. That we shouldn't eat.

JILL. But she does make delicious things. Anyway, the only thing Jessie said we needed to do was grab this. So I made a quick, painless trip and procured the necessary provisions.

(She holds up the plastic bag.)

NATHAN. No wine? She usually asks for wine.

JILL. We all drink wine. And she's bringing whatever she's bringing, so I was only, um, I was just supposed to provide these.

(She pulls two little plastic containers out of the bag.)

Tah dah.

NATHAN. What in the world?

JILL. It's some ginger. And this one is wasabi. I don't know why I said, "Tah dah" like it's magic. It's not magic. I got them from that sushi place off North Highland.

NATHAN. You got those from a chain restaurant?

> (**JILL** *is suddenly cautious. Like when you see*
> *a pit in the forest that someone has covered*
> *with leaves. Like when you see a trap.)*

JILL. I didn't make these little plastic containers, so yes.

NATHAN. Jill, you know how I feel about chain [restaurants.]

JILL. [And now you] understand why I didn't tell you I
    was going out. Look, Jessie said we needed ginger and
    wasabi and that's not something I usually shop for at
    the store, so I just went to the source.

NATHAN. It's the opposite of going to the source.

JILL. I swear to you, if you start in with one of your newly-
    minted slow food movement lectures, I [will scream.]

NATHAN. [I do not] lecture, I just want us to take better
    care of our bodies.

JILL. Then exercise.

NATHAN. I mean our insides.

JILL. Then take a probiotic.

NATHAN. Our souls.

JILL. Oh my god, Nathan, then go do some charity
    work. You're really going to die on this hill? "Take-out
    condiments" is the hill you want to die on?

> *(She shakes the condiments at him.)*

NATHAN. We could have gone to the Farmers' Market if
    you [had just...]

JILL. [I guess this] is the hill, I actually [might scream.]

NATHAN. [It's important to] me. And shopping at the
    Farmers' Market [is an...]

JILL. [For locally] grown wasabi? Locally grown wasabi from the local stream bed in a local Japanese mountain river valley?

NATHAN. You're trying to make it sound impossible.

JILL. I love you, now stop before [Jessie gets here and...]

NATHAN. [Come on, Jill, people] grow horseradish here and it's essentially the same thing [as wasabi.]

JILL. [It is not the] same thing, it's an entirely different plant. And Jessie said to have wasabi, specifically, so that's [what I...]

NATHAN. [When you] buy from some chain restaurant, [you're only...]

JILL. [No! No! No! No! Noooo!!]

(She cuts him off with a scream. Pause. She shrugs.)

NATHAN. Okay, yikes.

JILL. I told you I would scream.

NATHAN. We need to get better at communicating.

JILL. We're fine. We communicate fine.

NATHAN. Do we?

JILL. Look, I haven't seen Jessie in a while. So can we please just have a nice visit or whatever, and not bicker in front of her? Can we make that deal?

NATHAN. Fine. I get it.

JILL. Thank you. And after she leaves, maybe we can go to the Farmers' Market and take a leisurely stroll through the booths, okay?

NATHAN. Oh, you're appeasing me.

JILL. Does that count as slow food, if we walk slowly?

NATHAN. You're so funny.

JILL. You love it.

>   (*They kiss.*)

NATHAN. You taste like...you had a scone.

JILL. Don't be crazy.

NATHAN. You one hundred percent had a scone and it's blueberry. A scone or one of those muffins, admit it. Where did you buy the scone?

>   (*There's a knock.*)

JILL. Oh wow, Jessie's here.

>   (**JILL** *lets in* **JESSIE**. *She's smiling big. Bohemian chic. Carrying a plastic bag of something that looks a lot like fish guts. She throws her arms around* **JILL** *in a big hug. She does not look older than* **JILL**. *If anything she might even be younger.* **JILL** *and* **NATHAN** *are stunned.*)

JESSIE. It's so good to see you!

JILL. Jessie, you look...you look so...

JESSIE. What?

NATHAN. Good.

JILL. So good.

JESSIE. I know! Isn't it crazy?

JILL. But like, surgery good.

JESSIE. Okay, let's not.

JILL. No, I'm sorry, I don't think you had any work done. But...did you?

NATHAN. What did you do?

JESSIE. I'm just, ya know, living my life.

JILL. Jessie.

JESSIE. Really. All of the craziness on the news has really made me take stock, oh god, listen to me. I sound so fucking, no, you know what? I'm not going to judge it. I've been taking stock and trying to appreciate life more. You guys already had me on the road to health and all, so really [it's not...]

NATHAN. [But you] never listened to us.

JILL. Nathan.

NATHAN. She didn't.

JESSIE. I didn't.

JILL. But he doesn't have to say that.

JESSIE. It's okay, I tried. I really tried. And you guys have been so patient with me and now, well, just look.

JILL. It's uncanny. It's almost hypnotic. I can't stop looking at you.

JESSIE. Who says you have to?

JILL. You're practically glowing.

NATHAN. That's what it is; it's a glow.

JILL. I look like the older sister now.

JESSIE. Don't do that. Jill, I know we've been a little, teeny, tiny bit competitive in the past. Or I've been secretly competitive and you mostly just win, but all of that is behind us. Honestly. We can share this, especially because I brought a surprise for you!

(She holds out the plastic bag full of fish guts.)

NATHAN. Huh.

JESSIE. This is the secret. This is it.

> *(Pause. Then* **NATHAN** *and* **JILL** *laugh.* **JESSIE** *must be joking.)*

NATHAN. Very funny. You got us.

JILL. Here's a bag of bloody pulp. Surprise!

JESSIE. It is the surprise. Wait, is Mabel coming? Did you invite her?

JILL. I tried. She wasn't answering.

JESSIE. Fine. She misses out on the miracle.

> *(***JILL*** *does the bare minimum to mask her skepticism.)*

JILL. The plastic baggie miracle?

JESSIE. Yes, and I can hear the skepticism in your voice.

JILL. I wasn't really trying hard to hide it.

JESSIE. I know it looks gross. And I mean, some people are injecting it but that sounds, ugh, that sounds too intense. Overachievers, am I right? It's enough to just eat it. And you'll be amazed. Your skin will look better. You'll have more energy. The whole world really opens up, or at least that's my perception. And it only takes a bite. Here, take a little.

> *(She holds out the bag. They both reach in and smear a bit on their fingers. It looks gross and it looks like they think it's gross, too.)*

JILL. What's in it?

JESSIE. It's fish. It's the insides of the fish.

NATHAN. That's...not that bad. You like eating fish.

JILL. But what did the fish eat?

NATHAN. Smaller fish?

JILL. Jessie, you look amazing. I'm not discounting that there's obviously something at work here that's, I mean, amazing. But random fish don't suddenly become this kind of actual super food on their own. They eat something and it changes them then we eat them and it changes us.

NATHAN. Oh. Maybe it's just, maybe the omega-3 fatty acids are really strong?

JILL. Fatty acids don't make you look a decade younger.

JESSIE. A decade? Wow. Nice.

NATHAN. It was just a theory.

JILL. You don't have to know everything about everything.

NATHAN. I'm contributing.

JILL. Eat it if you want, no one's stopping you.

JESSIE. Jill, I can't believe I have to say this, but don't look a gift fish in the mouth.

JILL. I'm being open-minded.

(*She's not.*)

Just tell me where it came from.

NATHAN. That's a, that is a fair question, Jessie.

JESSIE. A small ice truck off Interstate 20. It comes once every two weeks. You should see the people waiting to buy, it's turning into some serious "Black Friday" action. This morning there was even some pushing and shoving. That was new. It's fine. Anyway, it's always the same two people. The one who drives the truck is a really kind lady. Oh, you'd laugh, Jill. She always has this little hat on with an enormous feather. Like, a single feather. I have no idea how she drives the truck wearing it.

NATHAN. She has a feather in her hat?

JILL. Sounds more like a fascinator.

JESSIE. It's a hat. And she has this real nervous energy, but she's nice enough. But the one who takes the money, this young guy, is really cute. He always wears these vintage T-shirts, or they look vintage. Great body.

JILL. So you buy the fish from weird strangers?

JESSIE. Do you know the guy who sells you fish at the supermarket by name?

JILL. Huh. And you just buy the fish whole off a truck?

JESSIE. What am I gonna gut my own fish? I don't understand why this is such a complicated idea. You pay for it, they gut the fish in front of you, and you take the insides just like this. You can also have the filets if you want. Or the heads, some people make soup or stock or something with the heads, I don't know. And the truck sells until it's empty, and then it drives away.

JILL. Drives where?

JESSIE. It drives, I don't know, just away. I guess back to wherever the magic fish swim. Jesus, Jill, it's a pinch of fish guts and your whole world changes.

JILL. You don't have to get offended.

JESSIE. I'm not offended. I'm annoyed. You're into this kind of stuff, right? You got me into this kind of stuff. You got me into Pilates, you got me into acupuncture, you got me to stop eating gluten, Nathan has me drinking coffee with butter in it and reading about this whole "slow food" thing.

NATHAN. Good for you.

JESSIE. I take twelve different probiotics, and you guys were right about all that. I'm just excited to contribute and finally be ahead of you on the curve for once. So sure, I'm being pushy. But it's not like I'm trying to get you to try black tar heroin. Honestly, the worst it could do is make you nauseous. The best thing is maybe you'll live forever. But I'm here to tell you it's actually just going to make you feel great. And, like you said, fucking "glow." Okay? So have we had enough of skeptical question time now?

> (**NATHAN** *eats his handful.* **JILL** *does too. It clearly doesn't taste good.*)

NATHAN. Done. Oh wow, it tastes terrible.

JESSIE. That's what the wasabi and ginger are for, but you guys went whole hog. Oh, and in case you were wondering, this doesn't have anything to do with all the weird, creepy stuff on the news about the lake. Like, I don't think any of this has to do with that lake stuff.

NATHAN. What lake stuff?

JESSIE. Seriously? You haven't seen the news lately?

JILL. We stopped watching because everything got so intense.

NATHAN. It didn't feel healthy anymore.

JESSIE. Sure. I hear that. Then just pretend I didn't say anything.

JILL. If there was some kind of warning then…

> (*Suddenly,* **NATHAN** *collapses to the ground.* **JILL** *abruptly collapses right after him. They both seem unconscious.*)

JESSIE. Just give it a second. It's rebuilding you from the inside out, but in a totally healthy way. It's all the good bacteria repopulating you. Just wait, you'll feel like entirely new people.

> (**JILL** *and* **NATHAN**'s *bodies shake on the floor in a burst, almost like seizures, and the lights flicker. Startled,* **JESSIE** *steps back. The bodies go still. After a moment,* **NATHAN** *and* **JILL**

get up, completely serene. They're calmer and happier than we've seen them at any point.)

JILL & NATHAN. Wow.

JESSIE. So? How do you feel?

JILL & NATHAN. Amazing.

JESSIE. So I was right?

JILL & NATHAN. Absolutely. I honestly haven't felt this good in years. Who knew gutting a fish could change everything just like that?

JESSIE. Just wait until it's done detoxifying your system. That's when the years really just start to fall off.

JESSIE, JILL & NATHAN. [And then you glow]

(They all smile. It's creepy.)

Five
1976

(CHARLIE is pacing in the "living room" of his studio apartment. He's in his underwear and a T-shirt. He is rehearsing a speech, but we can't make it out. Then there's a knock. He takes a breath and opens the door to DAN. He's in a winter coat and holding a bouquet of flowers.)

DAN. Hello!

(He's happy. CHARLIE's happy. DAN kisses CHARLIE. It is very welcome. Then he hands CHARLIE the bouquet of flowers.)

CHARLIE. Wow. Look at that. You brought me flowers?

DAN. Guilty. I saw them on the way over, I kind of want to pretend I planned it, but I just saw them and thought you'd like them. Or I don't know, I'm just in a mood. I was only gone for two weeks, but I missed you [so I just...]

CHARLIE. [That's super] sweet. They're great, Dan. Seriously. Oh, what is that?

(CHARLIE smells the flowers.)

DAN. Oh no. You don't love them.

CHARLIE. No, they're great. They just smell...strange.

(DAN smells them.)

DAN. Do they?

(They both smell the flowers again.)

I think they smell okay.

CHARLIE. It's me. It's totally me. I've been kind of out of it all week. My sinuses are acting up or something. They're great. The flowers are great. Thank you.

    *(He kisses **DAN**.)*

You look good. Is this a new jacket?

DAN. Charlie? Are you going to let me in?

CHARLIE. We can just go.

DAN. What? You're not even dressed.

CHARLIE. Right! I should get dressed. That is a thing people do, isn't it?

DAN. Are you okay? This is odd, even for you. Not odd. That sounds, no that's what I meant. It's fine. Take your time. We're not in a rush [or anything.]

CHARLIE. [Fuck, fuck, okay,] I have to tell you something.

DAN. I'm not even inside yet.

CHARLIE. Come in, I have to tell you something.

    *(**DAN** comes in and takes off his coat.)*

I was practicing what I want to say and I was gonna wait until later, but then, like, you showed up looking cute like you always do and gave me flowers and now I have to tell you.

DAN. That was quite a preamble.

CHARLIE. It's been a couple months and the bouquet of flowers is so nice [that I...]

DAN. [There really] isn't any, beyond "these are for you," there isn't any symbolism to the bouquet of flowers.

CHARLIE. Everything symbolizes something.

DAN. That idea makes me tired.

CHARLIE. There was this guy, last weekend there was this guy...

> (**CHARLIE** *stops. It's like he wants* **DAN** *to just get it.*)

DAN. Okay?

CHARLIE. There was this guy, and things got, I'm not seeing anyone else or anything, obviously since you and I are together, but you were gone and last weekend this guy, he...

> (**CHARLIE** *stops again. Still hoping* **DAN** *will get it.*)

DAN. I get it.

CHARLIE. Do you?

DAN. You totally fucked.

> (**DAN** *laughs at his own theory. But* **CHARLIE** *is massively relieved.*)

CHARLIE. Yes, we had sex. Yes, okay, I'm glad it's, like, out there.

DAN. What the fuck, Charlie, I was kidding? That was a joke guess!

CHARLIE. So I clearly didn't know that. I take it back.

DAN. You can't take it back. You fucked another guy?

CHARLIE. He fucked me, but it's super clear those logistics don't matter right now, and can we please forget that I said it? In fact it was joke, Dan! I was joking too because that's what we do, we joke.

DAN. Not okay.

CHARLIE. Of course it's not okay.

DAN. Not okay.

CHARLIE. Especially because of the flowers, when you show up with, but I mean, I'm not gonna look at your face and lie to you. And I thought you figured it out which was such a huge relief, but either way I had to tell you.

DAN. Why?

CHARLIE. Because we're supposed to be honest with the people we care about.

DAN. Gross.

CHARLIE. Gross?

DAN. Ugh, I really feel like once you've already broken the rules about how you're supposed to treat the people you care about you could be a little generous and just keep on breaking them to spare me a bit.

CHARLIE. Oh.

DAN. Yeah, "Oh."

CHARLIE. I just needed to tell you.

DAN. You really didn't.

CHARLIE. I guess, come on you know me, when something "feels" wrong I have to, like, address it.

DAN. I want to, I want to be calm and talk about, fuck, where's the bourbon?

> (**DAN** *looks for bourbon. He's doing his best not to rage out.*)

CHARLIE. Do you really want to drink right now?

DAN. I really want to drink right now instead of yelling.

CHARLIE. I'm trying to tell you it felt wrong to lie to you.

DAN. Just the lying part felt wrong?

CHARLIE. I didn't say that. But I'm sharing my truth with you.

DAN. Wow, aren't we all so perfectly self-actualized?

> *(He takes a swig directly from the bottle of bourbon.)*

CHARLIE. Drink as much as you want.

DAN. Oh, is that okay?

CHARLIE. I'm, I mean, okay, this is like, it's like how we took those personality tests, right? And mine said I'm a "Giver." Like that's the actual name of my personality [and I...]

DAN. [Oh my God, that] Myers-Briggs personality garbage is the same bullshit witchcraft that horoscopes are made of, can we please just not?

CHARLIE. I'm a Giver.

DAN. And I'm a Sagittarius.

CHARLIE. That personality test said I'm all about intuition and feeling. And I was overcome by this feeling, and I had to trust that, or it was kind of like I didn't have a choice on whether to trust it.

DAN. Do you know how that sounds?

CHARLIE. It sounds honest.

> *(**DAN** buckles down. He's really trying to understand where **CHARLIE** is coming from here. But he's hurt.)*

DAN. Huh. Okay. Okay, so if we were married, I'm not saying we're going to, if someday we were married for years and years and you had "a feeling" about another guy, then you'd have to honor that feeling?

CHARLIE. I don't know. In this scenario, am I still a "Giver" or [have I changed?]

DAN. [That personality test] also said you were ethical. Remember that part?

CHARLIE. I thought you weren't listening [when I...]

DAN. [I can think] it's dumb and still pay attention.

CHARLIE. I know you're upset. Be upset. Okay, I know I don't have to give you permission to be upset. But it's also, like, we never said we were strictly monogamous.

DAN. Huh.

CHARLIE. We never, like, codified it as a formal [kind of...]

DAN. [Codified it?]

CHARLIE. Is that not right? I'm saying we never sat down and had "the talk."

DAN. Sure. No, we never had "the talk."

CHARLIE. I guess that doesn't really make it better.

DAN. It's just very, I don't even know the word, it's... slippery? I know you're not a bad guy but it's still early in whatever this is and for that kind of thing to happen early, it's just all a little slippery, Charlie. And I sort of think you know it's slippery, I think you're sliding out of the handcuffs of your own confessional, like, "Hey, I did this bad thing, but it wasn't that bad because gray area." Okay, just... Okay, just tell me about the guy.

CHARLIE. What?

DAN. Tell me about [the guy.]

CHARLIE. [No, I'm not] [gonna...]

DAN. [If we're] being honest and feeling our feelings and really talking through, if we're processing this shit then I want to know about this guy you just couldn't resist. I'm waiting. I'm serious, I'll wait.

CHARLIE. I didn't think you'd [want to...]

DAN. [You didn't] think I'd ask about the guy?

CHARLIE. I thought it would be hard.

DAN. I thought we were in love.

CHARLIE. So did I until, like, right now. That's... What do you want to know?

DAN. I guess, just, whatever your "intuition" tells you to tell me.

CHARLIE. I don't know that much about him.

DAN. Fine. I'll give you prompts. Where did you meet?

CHARLIE. The Heretic.

DAN. You were at the Heretic?

CHARLIE. There was a party there for, whatever, it doesn't matter. Look, just because you don't like a place doesn't mean I have to stop going there.

DAN. What did he look like?

CHARLIE. He was my age, I think. Look, he was just a guy.

DAN. He was, huh, what was he wearing?

CHARLIE. Who cares? I'm [trying to...]

DAN. [I do, I] care. I care, okay?

CHARLIE. Okay, I get it. Um, I guess jeans. And a T-shirt that said "1976" on it, like a vintage shirt. Or it was supposed to look vintage. And he had...

(**CHARLIE** *stops again.*)

DAN. What?

CHARLIE. Never mind.

DAN. Charlie.

CHARLIE. It's not even a big thing. He just had one of those tattoos on his wrist.

DAN. So...?

CHARLIE. One of those sort of ribbon tattoos that wraps around. One of those, like, the ones the "lake" people get.

DAN. A tentacle?

CHARLIE. Is that what it is?

DAN. Fuck.

CHARLIE. See I wasn't gonna tell you because it's not a big deal.

DAN. You cheated on me with one of those weird culty zealots?

CHARLIE. He didn't seem like a zealot.

DAN. He had a tattoo. You don't think that's a little bit fanatical?

CHARLIE. He hardly said anything about the lake.

DAN. Fuck the lake.

CHARLIE. Shhh! I know you're mad, but don't, like, say that out loud.

DAN. Are you serious?

CHARLIE. Very. It's getting bigger. Like, the actual lake is getting bigger.

DAN. That doesn't make sense. And who even cares, there's no [one else here?]

CHARLIE. [Dan, Dan, listen, I've] seen some of the things they do now and maybe it's better to just [keep our...]

DAN. [Where? Where] did you see what they do?

CHARLIE. No, I'm saying that generally people [talk about...]

DAN. [What was the] party at the Heretic? It was a party, right? For what?

CHARLIE. I'm not allowed to talk about it.

DAN. You're not allowed?

CHARLIE. That's right.

*(Pause. **DAN** just stares at **CHARLIE**. Like he's never seen him.)*

Stop looking at me like that. Stop. Okay. Here's what I'll say. I shouldn't have gone to the party. I shouldn't have gone but I was curious, after all the stories, but then I saw what goes on, what they were doing, and I was wet and freaked out and felt dizzy and there was this smell and then he was just there, right in front of me, he was there and everything was kind of hazy, like when you're high, and he touched my face and I was looking at the numbers on his T-shirt and he told me to look down and I did and his pants were open some and then he looked at me and his eyes were, there was something in his eyes, like actually swimming around inside them, and he kissed me and it tasted like mud and wet grass and it was in the air and on his skin and then it was on my skin and I heard something in my ears from far away and then we had sex in front of everyone.

(Pause.)

DAN. That's so… Wait, in front of everyone? What were they doing? What were the other people there doing?

CHARLIE. I don't even know why he came up to me out of everyone there. I mean, I was terrified and freaked out, not looking to score [or whatever.]

DAN. [The other people,] what were they doing?

CHARLIE. They were watching us, they had these knives and hammers, no, don't think, I told you I'm not allowed to [talk about it.]

DAN. [Knives and] hammers?

CHARLIE. No, I didn't say that because I'm not talking about it.

DAN. You can intimately describe hooking up with another guy but you can't talk about what you saw at this party?

CHARLIE. It wasn't really a party, it was more like an, I don't know, a ritual?

DAN. That's not better!

CHARLIE. Can you smell that?

DAN. I don't smell anything? There isn't anything, there's nothing to smell.

CHARLIE. It smells like summer.

DAN. Okay. Listen, I'm trying to be open about this because you're being open and we've maybe really got something, or I [thought we did.]

CHARLIE. [I think so, too.]

DAN. But you recognize that this conversation keeps getting stranger and stranger. Not stranger, darker. I don't like it.

> (**CHARLIE** *suddenly tilts his head up a bit, staring into the middle distance. When he speaks, his voice is sweeter and joined by other voices. And those voices are doubled over and over, echoing around the room. It's not punctuated, it just happens. And it's unnerving.*)

CHARLIE + MULTITUDES. Everything would be lovely again if we just go to the lake.

DAN. How did you do that?

CHARLIE + MULTITUDES. Everything would be lovely again if we just go to the lake.

> (**CHARLIE** *picks up a knife off a nearby shelf, but then snaps out of it.*)

DAN. What the fuck?

CHARLIE. Why do you look like that?

(He looks down at the knife in his hand.)

Where did this [come from?]

DAN. [This is, huh,] this is not the right moment to fuck with me.

> *(**CHARLIE** tilts his head up a bit again, staring into the middle distance. When he speaks, his voice is sweeter and joined by other voices. And those voices are doubled over and over, echoing around the room. He moves between **DAN** and the door, brandishing the knife. He slowly starts approaching **DAN** while he speaks...)*

CHARLIE + MULTITUDES. Imagine how beautiful it would be to visit the lake. To walk just over the edge, just into the cool, dark water, and feel it caressing us. Shouldn't we go to the lake right now?

*(**CHARLIE** grabs **DAN** aggressively.)*

DAN. Charlie?!

*(**CHARLIE** snaps out of it and releases **DAN**. **DAN** leaps away.)*

CHARLIE. What?

DAN. What do you mean what?! You're talking crazy about the lake and pushing that damn knife against my throat! Keep back.

*(**CHARLIE** reflexively drops the knife.)*

CHARLIE. Dan, I didn't. I mean, I [wouldn't ever...]

DAN. [I'm going. Yeah,] fuck this, I'm gonna leave.

CHARLIE. Please don't. I don't know what's happening to me.

(**DAN** *grabs his coat and quickly puts it on.*)

DAN. Maybe it's the crazy voices or your new secret parties.

CHARLIE. This isn't, like, just please stay. I mean, I feel like this isn't something to break up over.

DAN. You feel wrong.

CHARLIE. I feel wrong?

DAN. I was... Jesus, Charlie, I was only gone for two weeks.

(**DAN** *exits.*)

CHARLIE + MULTITUDES. Goodbye.

Six
Lost Palace of The Butterfly King

(An open space. There is an enormous, illuminated screen in the back with a stylized shadow puppet landscape of mountains and rolling clouds. And butterflies flit around.)

*(The **BUTTERFLY KING** sits on the floor facing away upstage, legs crossed. He has no shirt and a beautiful pair of blue and black butterfly wings are tattooed on his back. He has a simple crown on his head.)*

(He shifts a bit to face out and reveal he is operating a pair of featureless marionettes, one with each hand. They are very old and have been crudely painted red. He acts out both roles.)

BUTTERFLY KING. "No, please! Please!"

"You have upset the Butterfly King."

"I didn't mean to, it was an accident!"

"Our God is not interested in your failings."

"It was only one basket of fish!"

"Half of everything must be left out for Him."

"But it's wasted food, it only rots."

"You dare question his volition?"

"What will you do to me?"

> *(The **BUTTERFLY KING** holds the "guilty" marionette up and grins.)*

You will be made an example.

(He slams the marionette on the floor over and over again causing the lights in the space to pulse and shake.)

(A **ZEALOT** *enters carrying a large, woven basket. It might have blood dripping from inside. She waits.)*

BUTTERFLY KING. What did you bring me?

(The **ZEALOT** *puts down the basket.)*

It isn't enough.

(The **ZEALOT** *leaves.)*

(The **BUTTERFLY KING** *returns to his marionettes.)*

"I heard that some worship a new God now."

"How when the Butterfly King is the only God?"

"People whisper of a new God beneath the water."

"And what does this new God say?"

"Nothing."

"How can they obey him if he says nothing?"

"It is a mystery."

(The **BUTTERFLY KING** *holds the "guilty" marionette up and grins.)*

You will be made an example.

(He slams the marionette on the floor over and over again causing the lights in the space to pulse and shake.)

(The **ZEALOT** *enters again carrying another large, woven basket. It might have blood dripping from inside. She sets it down.)*

It is never enough!

(**MABEL** *enters. She is carrying her small plate of cake from earlier and a fork. She is still eating as she takes in the space.*)

MABEL. Excuse me. I'm sorry to bother you, but do you know where I am?

(*The* **ZEALOT** *leaves.*)

All right then.

BUTTERFLY KING. Who are you?

MABEL. I'm Mabel. I made this poison cake and then I waited outside in a really long line and now I'm here.

BUTTERFLY KING. If it's poison, stop eating it.

MABEL. You're right, that sounds right. But it never runs out, I've been eating it in line this whole time. There's just always cake.

(*She takes another bite.*)

BUTTERFLY KING. Stop eating it.

MABEL. Of course, you're right.

(*She takes another bite.*)

BUTTERFLY KING. And that is why you're here.

MABEL. Because of the cake?

BUTTERFLY KING. Because you killed yourself and people who kill themselves come to me.

MABEL. Here?

BUTTERFLY KING. Yes.

MABEL. Is this Hell?

BUTTERFLY KING. No. You're adorable.

MABEL. Where is it?

BUTTERFLY KING. My palace.

> *(He waves his hand and the shadows behind
> him shift to reveal an enormous palace on the
> side of a mountain.)*

MABEL. So I'm dead?

BUTTERFLY KING. You poisoned yourself.

MABEL. I was scared.

BUTTERFLY KING. You also poisoned two other people.

MABEL. I spared them from the suffering I saw coming.

BUTTERFLY KING. Did you?

MABEL. They didn't have to come to my house and eat
my cake.

BUTTERFLY KING. All the same.

MABEL. I don't want to think about it.

BUTTERFLY KING. That's healthy.

> *(She takes another bite and looks around.)*

MABEL. Hmmm.

BUTTERFLY KING. "Hmmm," what?

MABEL. Oh, I just...thought it would be different. Whatever's
on the other side, if this is really the other side.

BUTTERFLY KING. You don't believe me?

MABEL. It's just a lot to take in. And honestly, it's a little
hard to, well, I'm supposed to believe some guy on the
floor playing with puppets?

> *(He laughs and it is big and manic. Mocking.
> Then he announces...)*

BUTTERFLY KING. "Some guy"? I am one thousand Blue Moon butterflies wearing a crown.

MABEL. Yes, well...well, I don't know how to respond to that.

> *(The **BUTTERFLY KING** drops all of his royal grandeur.)*

BUTTERFLY KING. I am the Butterfly King. And now you belong to me.

MABEL. Excuse me, I belong to you?

BUTTERFLY KING. You're my guest.

MABEL. That's different.

BUTTERFLY KING. Forever.

> *(Pause.)*

MABEL. You're being very accommodating, but you're saying some crazy things.

BUTTERFLY KING. You filled a cake full of a lethal plant and ate it because you were feeling anxious, and I'm crazy?

MABEL. How did you know about the foxglove?

> *(The **BUTTERFLY KING** takes the marionettes and acts out a moment...)*

BUTTERFLY KING. "Why did you burn your things?"

"Because nothing means anything anymore."

"Oh wow."

"I told you it was bleak. And then I baked this cake. [With a lot...?]"

MABEL. "[With a lot] of foxglove. Do you know it?" That's uncanny. And I can't deny that it's me.

(The **BUTTERFLY KING** *holds the marionette up and grins at* **MABEL.***)*

BUTTERFLY KING. You will be made an example.

MABEL. Well, I suppose I don't have a choice at this point.

BUTTERFLY KING. I mean, you already waited in line.

(He waves his hand again revealing a long line of people that wraps from the palace around the mountain and off to the horizon. She looks at the line, then she looks around the palace.)

MABEL. All right. All right. Honestly, I accept this. I accept it. I feel okay about it.

BUTTERFLY KING. Good for you.

MABEL. It's so much better than what I left behind. I just could not abide what was happening to people. And that thing in the lake? I don't want to be in a world where that thing in the lake exists.

BUTTERFLY KING. It's just another very old thing. In fact, we're old friends.

MABEL. It's making people do bad things.

BUTTERFLY KING. "Bad things?" Good and bad belong in children's storybooks.

MABEL. It's making people do "horrible" things.

BUTTERFLY KING. Is it now?

(He operates the marionettes, but focuses on **MABEL.***)*

"How's your cake?"

"It's delicious."

MABEL. It is delicious, I make delicious things.

BUTTERFLY KING. Mabel, I think you'll find that people don't really need to be made to do horrible things. In fact, I think you'll find that many people are just looking for a reason to do horrible things. And as soon as that reason comes along, off they go to do the things that would shock you.

MABEL. That's very dark.

BUTTERFLY KING. I didn't say all people.

(He holds up one of the marionettes and makes it wave.)

Some people are perfectly nice.

(Then he abruptly slams the marionette on the floor over and over again causing the lights in the space to pulse and shake.)

*(**MABEL** is startled and drops her plate.)*

Oh no, you dropped your cake.

MABEL. I was startled. You startled me.

BUTTERFLY KING. Such a shame.

MABEL. You told me to stop eating it.

BUTTERFLY KING. If you get hungry later, we'll find something for you to eat.

*(**MABEL** sits on the floor across from the **BUTTERFLY KING.**)*

MABEL. Are you...what are you?

BUTTERFLY KING. Oh that's fun. What am I?

MABEL. That's right.

BUTTERFLY KING. What is a living thing? What is a life?

MABEL. There's no need to be grand.

BUTTERFLY KING. Grand?

(He laughs.)

MABEL. Yes. Grand.

BUTTERFLY KING. I like you, Mabel. All right, what am I? Well, I already told you that I am "one thousand Blue Moon butterflies wearing a crown." But I think you mean your question in a more existential sense. So I suppose I'm just one more very old thing.

> *(The **ZEALOT** enters again carrying another large, woven basket. It might have blood dripping from inside. She sets it with the others.)*

> *(The **ZEALOT** leaves.)*

MABEL. Well… I'm sorry to say it, but I've never heard of you.

BUTTERFLY KING. You'd be amazed what you've never heard of in your life.

MABEL. Oh no, I meant that no one's ever heard of you.

BUTTERFLY KING. That's a very broad generalization.

MABEL. I'm being very sincere with you, Mr. Butterfly King.

BUTTERFLY KING. Then why do people keep killing themselves for me?

MABEL. They're not.

BUTTERFLY KING. Then why do they do it?

MABEL. All sort of reasons, sadness, illness, rage, because the world is too much of all those things or not enough of them. But I'm almost one hundred percent sure that no one is committing suicide as a tribute to some mythic Butterfly King.

BUTTERFLY KING. Mythic in a "grand" way?

MABEL. Did you think people were killing themselves for you?

BUTTERFLY KING. As it happens, I did. I really did. I mean, they certainly used to.

MABEL. Did they?

BUTTERFLY KING. Oh, yes. They used to kill themselves, their neighbors, their loved ones, all for me. They used to light bonfires, they used to consume each other's flesh, such fun.

MABEL. Oh no.

BUTTERFLY KING. This is very disappointing.

MABEL. Oh.

BUTTERFLY KING. I'm so disappointed.

MABEL. I'm not really sorry, but I'll say it if that will help?

*(The **ZEALOT** enters again carrying another large, woven basket. It might have blood dripping from inside. She sets it down and leaves.)*

BUTTERFLY KING. If no one is killing themselves or each other for me anymore, then where does this keep coming from?

MABEL. What is that?

BUTTERFLY KING. Tributes.

MABEL. Is that blood leaking out of the baskets?

BUTTERFLY KING. So no one knows about me, but they believe in the thing in the lake?

MABEL. They're beginning to believe in it, yes.

BUTTERFLY KING. Ugh, people are so fickle.

(Pause. They sit in an awkward silence.)

MABEL. So I'm here forever now?

BUTTERFLY KING. It won't feel like forever. You'll lose little bits of yourself over time and one day it will be like you were always here and we'll all just keep moving forward together.

MABEL. Moving forward towards…what?

BUTTERFLY KING. Oh, I'm being rude. You must be hungry again.

MABEL. All right, I think…I think maybe I shouldn't have done this.

BUTTERFLY KING. Are you hungry?

MABEL. I should not have done this. I shouldn't have done this. Isn't that something? Huh, I feel so hollow all of the sudden.

BUTTERFLY KING. But are you hungry?

MABEL. Is that what it is? I don't know.

> (*The* **BUTTERFLY KING** *gets up for the first time, goes to the baskets and opens one. He looks down into it, reaches inside, and pulls out a handful of something red, wet, and fleshy. He replaces the lid and walks over to* **MABEL**. *He tears off a piece and hands it to her.*)

BUTTERFLY KING. I don't mind sharing.

> (*She takes it. He sits back down across from her.*)

MABEL. Thank you. Oh, but do we have time to just sit and eat?

BUTTERFLY KING. So much time.

MABEL. It's just that there are so many people waiting in that long line outside.

(He waves his hand and the images of clouds return, obscuring the palace and the endless line of people.)

BUTTERFLY KING. Like you said, none of them believe in me anymore. Let them wait.

(The **BUTTERFLY KING** *and* **MABEL** *eat.)*

Seven
Liturgical Dances

(Back in the living room of the lake house. **ALEX** *and* **RYAN** *sit on the couch pulling papers out of a box, looking through the old files and printouts for something specific. Other boxes litter the mostly empty room.)*

ALEX. I just don't understand why they need all of this stuff.

RYAN. Because my mom left me this lake house, which is all fine and good. But in order to actually sell it we need to give them everything.

ALEX. Then let's just give them everything.

RYAN. The whole box of documents?

ALEX. Yep.

RYAN. There's a lot of important stuff in here.

ALEX. So important it's been in the attic for a thousand years.

RYAN. I don't know. Maybe. Going through it all, we find out.

ALEX. That's fair.

(She stops and takes him in as he continues to dig through the box.)

Okay, do you think the missing papers are a sign? Like the universe is telling us not to leave?

RYAN. The universe?

ALEX. Stop it, you know what I mean.

RYAN. This box is a sign that my mom, God rest her soul, was really bad at keeping her affairs in order. I don't think it has any deeper meaning.

(Music starts up somewhere outside.* It's close enough to hear, but not right on top of them. They both turn to look towards the lake. They look at each other, a tense moment. Then...)

ALEX. Okay. Okay, your mom was disorganized, and we need the deed and mortgage papers, that's good enough for me. Let's find those papers.

RYAN. Great. Do you want to start looking in that box? I'll keep working on this one. But I, it's a little crazy, but I do still want to know what actually goes on down there at the lake.

ALEX. Ryan, not [this again.]

RYAN. [You really] don't? Not even a little bit?

ALEX. Not even a little bit. And I don't know why you keep bringing it up.

RYAN. Alex.

ALEX. I don't want to know any of it. I've seen the videos, I hear them yelling and shouting by the lake, I hear the music and the screams, the cheering. And that's all I need to know. It already feels like, no, never mind.

RYAN. It already feels like what?

ALEX. You're gonna think I'm being paranoid.

RYAN. I won't. In fact, I promise not to react. How about that?

ALEX. Okay. Okay, look, I understand geography and what I'm about to say is very strange. But it feels like the lake is closer to us now. Like, physically.

---

* A license to produce *Sleeping Giant* does not include a performance license for any third-party or copyrighted music. Licensees should create an original composition or use music in the public domain. For further information, please see the Music and Third-Party Materials Use Note on page iii.

*(She points outside. **RYAN** grins but quickly covers his mouth.)*

RYAN. No, sorry.

ALEX. You said you wouldn't, don't grin like that, I'm serious.

RYAN. I tried. But it's not closer. It's a lake. It's not following [us or anything.]

ALEX. [That's not what] I, okay, I meant that it was bigger.

RYAN. I think you're freaked out and your brain is playing tricks on you.

ALEX. You really haven't noticed?

RYAN. I really haven't.

(She starts pacing. She's clearly anxious but trying to not to show it.)

ALEX. Okay. Maybe you're right. I hope you're right. We can disagree about it later in the car when we're far away from this town.

RYAN. If you're so amped to get on the road, why did you think the universe was giving us a sign to stay?

ALEX. Oh my god, I didn't. I just wanted to give you an out in case you didn't really want to sell the place. This house is a lot to give up. I mean sure, I could probably keep living here and just "not know" what goes on down at that lake. But that sounds sad. To live in, like, willful ignorance.

RYAN. I'm not asking you to, no one is asking. And I'm not even sure there's even anything in the lake anyway, all of this [might just be...]

*(She turns her entire focus to **RYAN**...)*

ALEX. [Stop it.]

RYAN. No, think about it. Have you seen it? With your own eyes?

ALEX. What does that prove? I've never experienced the vacuum of space, but I know it's not good. I've never fallen off a cliff, but I know I wouldn't like it. I've never been caving, but I know that I'd get stuck in one of those small passages and suffocate alone underground in the dark.

RYAN. Whoa.

ALEX. I've never seen a horrifying giant squid, but they exist.

RYAN. This list is insane.

ALEX. So is a fucking lake monster. You don't have to experience something firsthand to be afraid of it. And maybe I'm a little more worked up than I normally would be because it's pretty much our fault this is happening.

RYAN. How is this our fault?

ALEX. Ryan. You know it was those fucking fireworks from the proposal that woke it up [in the first place.]

RYAN. [How many times do] I need to apologize [for the fireworks?]

ALEX. [And now this "thing" is] making [people strange.]

RYAN. [You said they were] a little bit beautiful.

ALEX. Something can be beautiful and still cause bad things to happen.

RYAN. It's not our fault.

ALEX. Seems like it is though.

RYAN. Fine. Agree to disagree.

> *(He returns to looking through the papers again.)*

ALEX. Okay, how about what happened with Billy? He [was terrified.]

RYAN. [It really wasn't] a big deal. Billy was just spooked, and [we were too.]

ALEX. [Billy literally] opened his mouth and the very loud sound of some kind of pagan primordial horror came out.

RYAN. Have you been reading my Butterfly King book?

ALEX. Some. Enough to know that's not a past I have any interest in repeating.

RYAN. I don't think we're in danger of repeating that specifically gruesome past.

ALEX. Okay well, whatever they're doing down there at the lake, it's probably a lot like whatever all those Pacific Islanders were doing right before they started eating each other and killing themselves for the Butterfly King.

RYAN. And that's exactly why I want to see for myself.

ALEX. Jesus. It's mind-bending how none of this is getting through to you.

RYAN. Just, I'm not convinced we really heard what we heard when Billy was here. We were fuzzy from the fireworks and the smoke, [and Billy was...]

ALEX. [So you're saying] you do want to keep the house.

RYAN. Oh my god, no. I'm just saying I'm curious.

ALEX. Are you, huh, are you losing your mind? Is everyone losing their minds? Honestly, we should have told people that first night. We should have tried to stop it, but it's too big to stop now.

RYAN. How were we supposed to stop all of this?

ALEX. We could have taken Billy to the police and told them Mike was missing. We could have gone to the local paper and reported it.

RYAN. "Lake monster scares teenage boy."

ALEX. "Lake monster kills teenage boy." Have you seen Mike since that night? We used to see him almost every day, fishing or boating. Have you seen him anywhere since that night?

> *(Pause.)*

RYAN. No.

ALEX. And that's fine? That's just how things are around here now?

RYAN. That's why we're selling the house. Okay? Alex, like I said, I was just curious. But you are more important than solving the mystery of the lake. Once we find these papers for the bank we are gone.

> *(He takes her hand. She nods "Okay" and then...)*

ALEX. Can we please leave your mother's old mattress here?

RYAN. Absolutely.

> *(There's a chipper knock at the door. They exchange a look.)*

ALEX. Okay. It's pretty late for someone to just, like, drop by.

> *(**ALEX** opens the door and **BILLY** and **BARBARA** walk right in. He's in jeans and the same "1976" T-shirt. He has a tattoo around his wrist of a tentacle. She's in a new variation on her earlier outfit, complete with a brand-new fascinator, still sporting her tight smile. The fascinator has a single, even larger feather.)*

BILLY. Hello again!

BARBARA. We don't have time for this.

BILLY. It will only take a minute.

ALEX. Oh! Billy, hey. Hey, how [are you?]

> *(Everyone is smiling, but no one is really relaxed or casual. And* **BARBARA** *is as anxious as ever.)*

> *(Water also begins to slowly seep into the room from the lake outside. It's coming from the same direction* **BILLY** *and* **BARBARA** *entered. Like it's following them. None of them acknowledge the water, even as it moves underfoot.)*

BILLY. [We were on] our way down to the lake and I saw the "For Sale" sign. You're moving?

RYAN. Oh, yes. We are. This was my mom's place and there's just, you know, too many memories.

BILLY. But you're right in the heart of something so special.

ALEX. We know. It's such a shame to have to leave.

BILLY. But you're right in the heart of something so special.

RYAN. You already said that.

BILLY. I never got to apologize to you, for probably completely creeping you out the night of the fireworks. It's been a while, but do you remember?

RYAN. It was definitely an odd night.

BILLY. I was so out of it, right? Thanks for looking out for me. I wanted Barbara to meet you, too. Oh, this is Barbara. She's become a huge volunteer.

BARBARA. We're going to be late.

ALEX. I love your hat.

BARBARA. It's not a hat!!!

(Awkward pause.)

ALEX. Sorry.

BARBARA. No, I'm sorry. But it's a fascinator. I'm just sensitive about it.

RYAN. What are you volunteering for?

BILLY. You're right in the heart of something so special.

ALEX. Okay.

BARBARA. If you're going to ask them, then ask them.

BILLY. We'd love for you to come down to the lake tonight.

ALEX. We're packing! We're, um, we have to pack things up.

RYAN. My family's owned this place for a long time, so it's a lot to get through.

BARBARA. Wait a minute. Wait, do they not want to come to the lake? Do you not want to come to the lake?

RYAN. Of course [we do.]

ALEX. [We've tried] to make it, we're [just always…]

BARBARA. [Are you] lying?

BILLY. Now Barbara, Alex and Ryan wouldn't lie to us. Maybe they're just intimidated when it comes to trying new things.

ALEX. No, just busy. So busy.

RYAN. But since you brought it up, maybe you could explain [to us what…]

ALEX. [Ryan, we] don't want to keep them.

BILLY. I don't mind. Unless you'd like to explain, Barbara?

BARBARA. Eyeball.

BILLY. Then I'll do it. Everyone gathers on the shore of the lake, just in the water. We take our shoes off, of course. And then we dance. There's music and we dance.

BILLY. It can last for hours and it's so joyous. Some people even glow. And then the first person to stop dancing is sacrificed to the lake. That lucky person is cut and drowned and given to the water so that the rest of us can have happiness and good health. And then we start again. We can do two or three a night, depending on our numbers. That's why it's so important to have new believers. Simple as that.

> (*Pause. Everyone is smiling. Nodding. Simple. The water spilling in now covers the living room floor.*)

RYAN. That's...really something. Happiness and good health are the goal. That's something. Isn't it, honey?

ALEX. Yes.

BILLY & BARBARA. The God in the lake grants us both in abundance.

RYAN. Sounds great.

ALEX. Super great.

BILLY. So you'll come?

RYAN. As soon as we get moved, we will definitely come check it out.

BILLY. So you'll come tonight?

ALEX. We already told you [that we...]

BILLY. [My parents will] be there tonight and most of the neighbors around the lake, people from town, some police officers, some teachers, even some children, along with so many new people to meet.

BARBARA. The people are amazing. And waiting for us.

> (**BILLY** *doesn't look away from* **ALEX** *and* **RYAN**.)

BILLY. We'll go soon.

RYAN. Look, Billy... We just, we won't be there tonight. I'm sorry, but we can't. So thank you again for the invitation and it was such a treat to meet you Barbara. So you can go ahead now. Can I show you out?

BILLY. I know the way.

> (**BILLY** and **BARBARA** start to leave. Suddenly, **BILLY** turns back. **BARBARA** reluctantly waits, but she's clearly annoyed.)

One last thing, you know the McAllisters, right?

ALEX. Dana and Rob, sure.

RYAN. From four houses down.

ALEX. They've been out of town, I think.

BILLY. Well, Dana and Rob didn't want to come last week. They were busy. Everyone's so busy, right? And when I told everyone at the lake that they were too busy, people just didn't understand. So everyone went to the McAllister's house together and convinced them to come participate. Of course, by the time they were convinced they were too hurt to dance very long and Rob ended up in the water.

ALEX. Are you saying that Rob is... Are you saying that you killed...?

BILLY. I'm saying Dana is a more dedicated dancer.

> (Pause.)

And I think it would be a shame if people had the same reaction to the news about you being so busy. Honestly, they just want the God in the lake to be happy. And satisfied. That's all.

RYAN. We'll be there shortly.

ALEX. Ryan.

RYAN. It's fine, honey. We can make the time. We will wrap things up here and come right down. Sound good to you two?

BARBARA. Sounds wonderful.

BILLY. It does sound wonderful, doesn't it? It sounds like a whole new world.

BARBARA. Ready?

> *(Suddenly, everything goes dark as pink specials zero in on* **BARBARA**. *This time* **BILLY** *is included. Lights undulate on them, oily and odd.)*

> *(***BILLY*** looks up, basking in the light.* **BARBARA** *opens her mouth to sing, but suddenly her voice comes from somewhere else, many different versions of her voice, in a loud overlapping cluster of "Three Blind Mice" with dozens of people eerily whistling the tune at different speeds. It just keeps growing into a jarring cacophony.)*

> *(***BARBARA*** was clearly not expecting it. What even is this?* **BILLY** *looks peaceful, but* **BARBARA** *panics, covering her ears and crying. She begins screaming over the sound...)*

Why are they, why are they blind?! What happened to their eyes?! Where are their eyes?! Where the fuck are their eyes?!

> *(Then abruptly the lights shift back to normal and it all resumes.* **BARBARA** *pulls herself back together but is still kind of freaking out.)*

That's enough of this. We have to go; I have to go right now.

(She rushes out the door.)

BILLY. Wow. You know, it really is a calling for her. We should all be so lucky to find that kind of joy in our lives. Doesn't she seem joyful? Oh, that reminds me, most of the streets out of town are blocked. There are just so many people trying to get to the lake. I guess it's good you've decided to stay. So we'll see you down there. Shortly.

> *(**ALEX** and **RYAN** smile and nod. **BILLY** finally leaves. And the minute he goes, the water begins flooding into the room even faster. **ALEX** and **RYAN** stop smiling. They are desperate.)*

ALEX. This is not... Okay, we are not...?

> *(Suddenly, the music gets louder. It's coming from the lake. People must be dancing. They both turn to look towards the door. Then they look down at the lake literally spilling into their house.)*

RYAN. Oh god.

ALEX. Ryan. They killed Rob McAllister and fed him to a fucking lake monster.

RYAN. This can't be real.

ALEX. It doesn't matter, Ryan. It doesn't matter if it's real! They think it's real and they murdered Rob. And where is Dana? She hasn't been back to their house; we would have seen her. Is she dead too? Two or three people a night, he said. They are killing [two or three...]

RYAN. [Maybe she's just] hiding. With the lights out, maybe [she's in her...]

ALEX. [Jesus, she's not] hiding. Oh my god, what are we [going to do?]

RYAN. [We were] leaving. We're still going to leave.

ALEX. You heard him, we're trapped here tonight.

RYAN. Then I don't know, Alex.

> *(The music stops abruptly. They look towards the lake as water continues to spill inside. Suddenly the sound of horrified screaming, like someone being brutally killed. The screaming is quickly swallowed up by raucous cheering. Then the music starts again.)*

> *(**RYAN** and **ALEX** look at each other. They are terrified.)*

ALEX. It's too late.

RYAN. How...how is your dancing?

End of Play